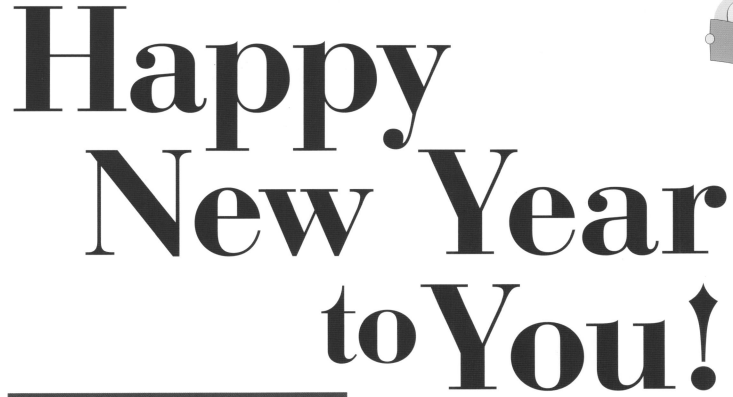

A TWO-LAP BOOK™

Happy New Year to You!

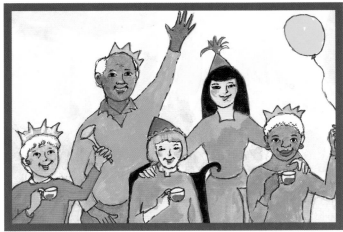

**A Read-Aloud Book for
Memory-Challenged Adults**

by Lydia Burdick
ILLUSTRATED BY JANE FREEMAN

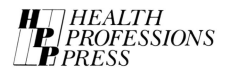

HEALTH
PROFESSIONS
PRESS

Baltimore • London • Sydney

In loving memory of my parents, Shirley and Larry Burdick

And treasured family and friends—

Ida and Isidore Burdick and Irma and Leopold Gross

Gert and Bob Bodner and Sam Rosenberg

Lucille and Sidney Burdick, Rudolph Gross, and Lee Bloch

Angelina Pacheco, Stewart Mahana, Brendan Sirlin, and
Michael Steuerman

I also dedicate this book to—

The professionals who continue with open minds to look for the
causes of Alzheimer's disease and other dementias and for how to
prevent them. My appreciation goes to health care practitioners
and researchers in allopathic medicine, biological medicine,
complementary medicine, environmental medicine, biological
dentistry, nutrition, and toxicology.

My wonderful partners at Health Professions Press—it is a joy to
work and create with you.

My friend and illustrator extraordinaire, Jane Freeman—your
glorious art brings my words to rich and vibrant life.

And most importantly to you, Dear Reader, and the loved ones
you are caring for and reading with.

—Lydia Burdick

To Joe and Jory, with my love.

—Jane Freeman

From the Author

There is something intimate and magical about reading a book together. You can savor this pleasure when you read *Happy New Year to You!* with a loved one who has memory loss.

Two-Lap Books™ are designed for intimacy; the books are large enough to be spread across two laps. They are written and illustrated to relate to most people's lives—present and past.

I wrote the first book in this series, *The Sunshine on My Face*, for my mother, Shirley Burdick, who was diagnosed with Alzheimer's disease. I wanted to give her words to say and pictures to look at that related to her life as it was at the time. I also wanted to give us a happy activity to do together. My goal was to see a smile on her face with every page.

When I sat down that first time with my mother and with the materials that would become *The Sunshine on My Face*, I didn't know if she would read these sentences to herself, out loud to me, or at all. My mother had been answering our questions only in monosyllables for some time and did not initiate any conversation on her own.

To my delight, with gentle prompting and encouragement, my mother read all the words I presented to her, out loud. There was recognition and pleasure in her voice and bigger smiles than I had seen in years. My written words and the illustrations served as a bridge between us. I had achieved my goal!

I have been thrilled to hear from so many family and professional caregivers about the joyful experiences they have had reading *The Sunshine on My Face* with loved ones, patients, and clients who have memory loss. I hope that *Happy New Year to You!*, the latest book in the Two-Lap Books™ series, will provide you and your reading partner with similar wonderful rewards.

—Lydia Burdick

How to Use This Book

GETTING STARTED

Tell your reading partner that you have a book you think he or she will enjoy. Get comfortable together. Sit close enough for the book to cover both of your laps. If this is not possible, position yourselves so the book is easily accessible for both of you.

READING TOGETHER

If you think your companion is able to read, invite him or her to read the words to you. You might say, "Mom, I'd love you to read this page to me" or "Mr. Smith, I'll read this page and you read the next, okay?" If you don't get a positive response, be patient. Ask the person to read a few times, always with a smile and without any pressure. It might take awhile for the other person to get involved in the activity—be encouraging.

You can read the words out loud together. If your partner does not wish to read or is not able to read, then read the book out loud to him or her.

You can read this book together from cover to cover several times, read it through once, read a few favorite pages, or read just one page—whatever you and your reading companion choose to do.

Talk with your partner about the sentences. Ask simple questions about the pictures and the themes. How do they relate to life today or in the past? You will find **conversation prompts** at the end of the book.

You can also read the book as a group activity, taking turns reading the content and asking questions about it.

LOOKING AT THE ILLUSTRATIONS

Take time to enjoy the pictures and talk about what you see. Sometimes you may want to talk about the pictures alone, without reading the text.

SINGING TOGETHER

Singing is a wonderful activity that triggers happy memories and brings people together. Many songs are brought to mind by the pictures, actions, and seasons on each page. Some **suggested songs for each month** are provided with the conversation prompts at the end of the book. Sing the songs you enjoy and bring music into this activity.

PLAYING GAMES

Many characters and objects repeat in the pictures. Play the game "find the dog," for example, for each month of the year.

READING LONG-DISTANCE

You and your reading partner can read a Two-Lap Book™ out loud over the phone to a family member or friend. It can be a thrill from long distance to hear the voice of a loved one when he or she has mostly stopped talking.

ENJOYING YOUR TIME TOGETHER

Let this book be the spark for an enjoyable and meaningful time together.

Happy reading!

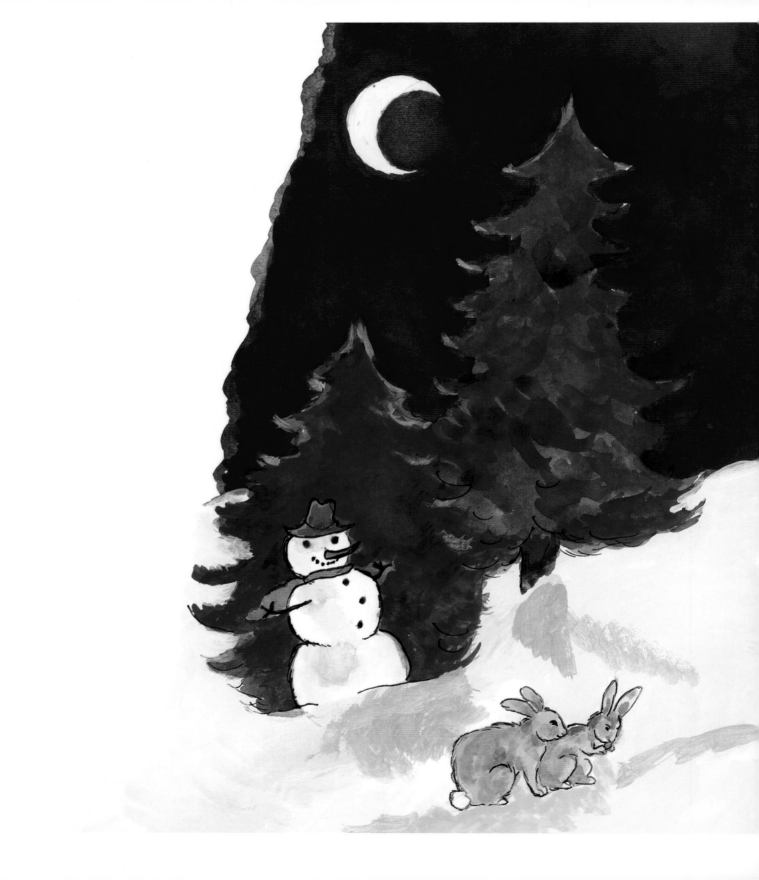

In January I wish you "Happy New Year!"

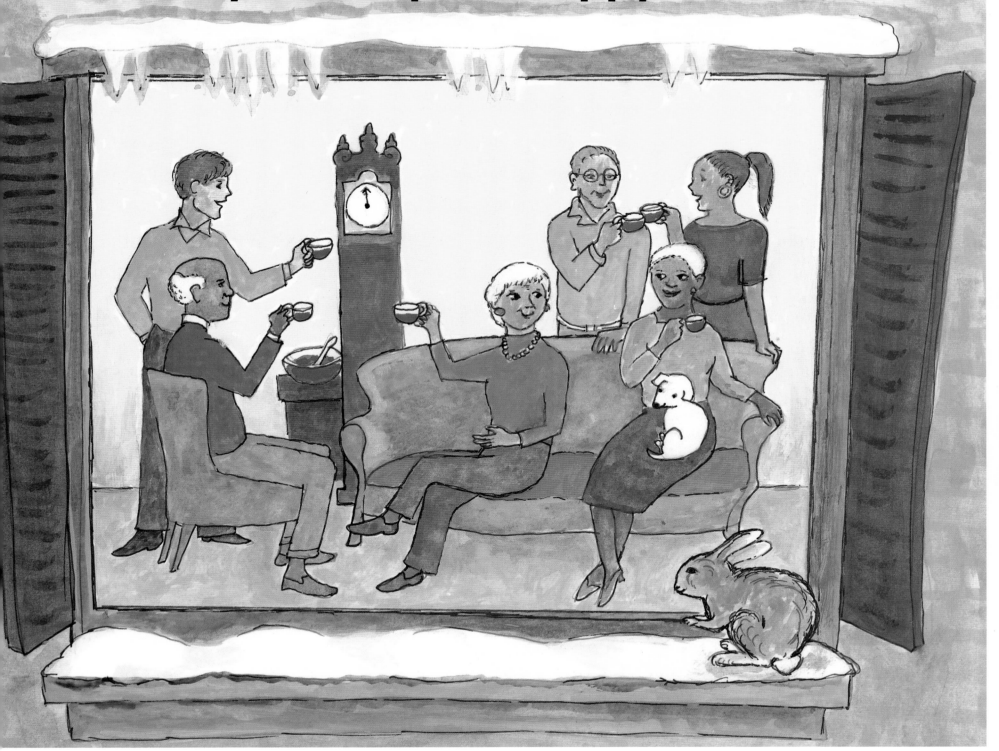

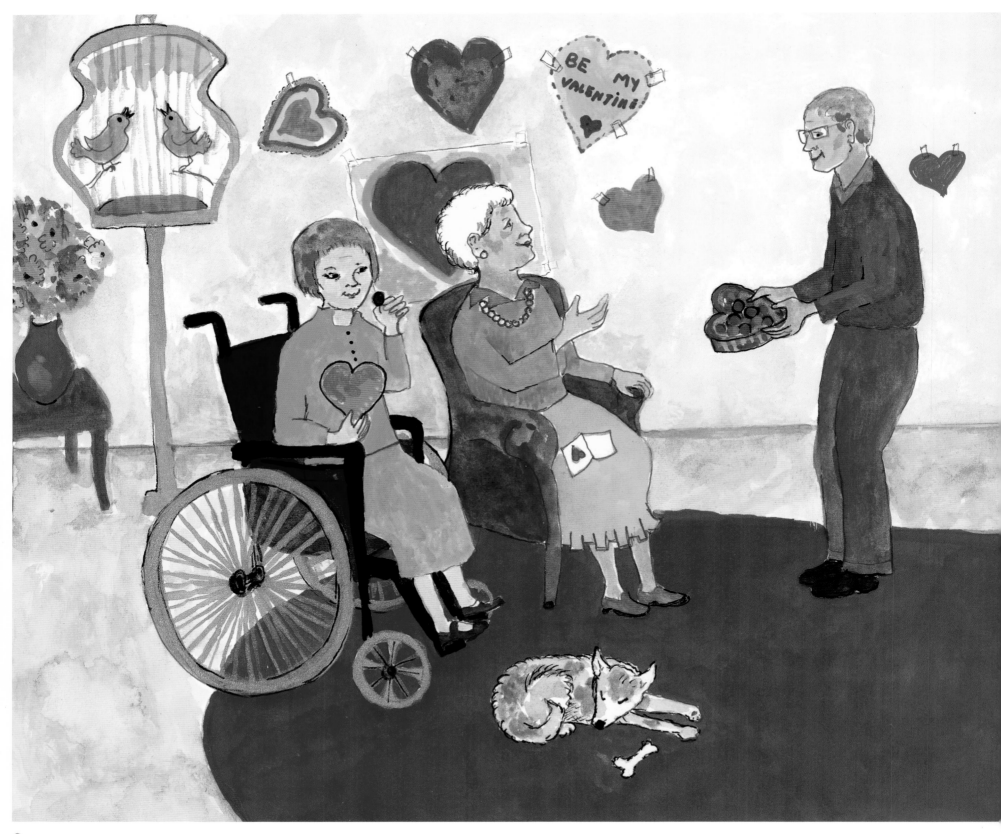

In February
will you be my Valentine?

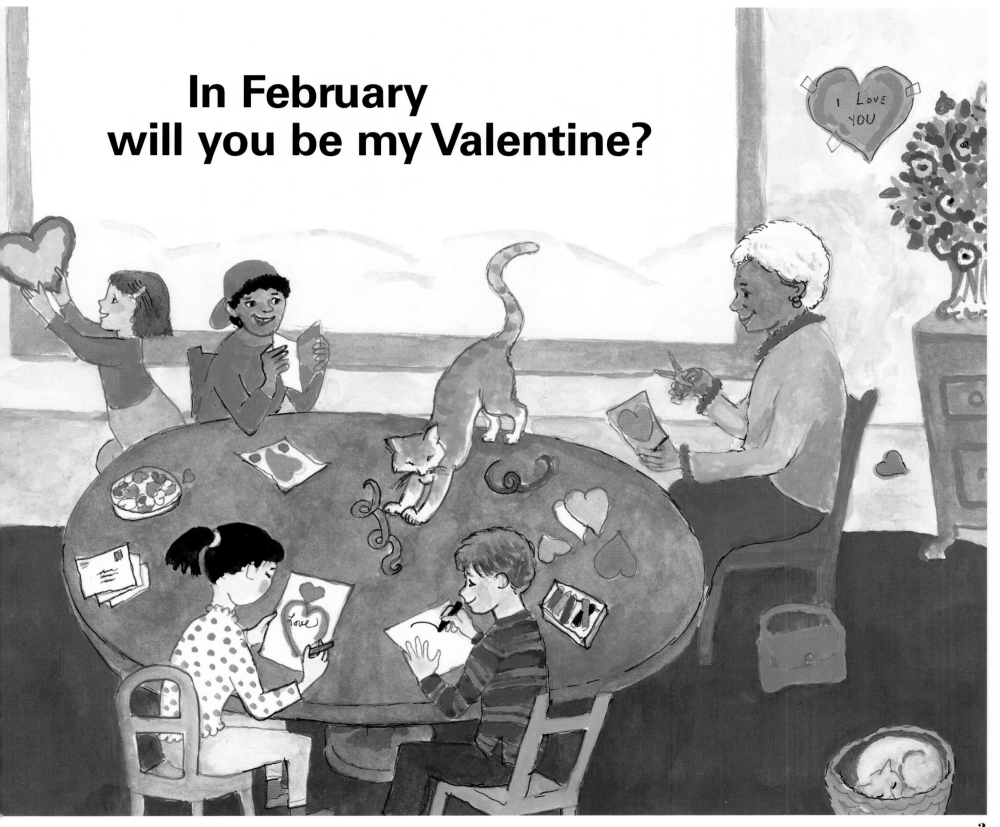

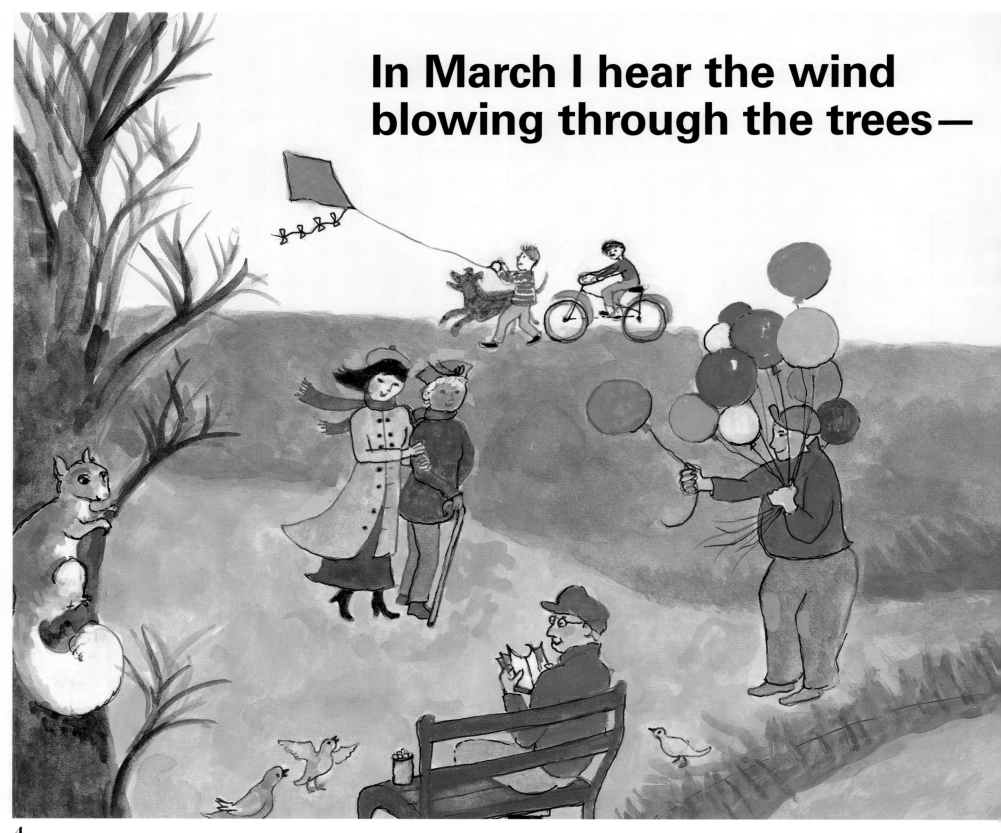

In March I hear the wind blowing through the trees—

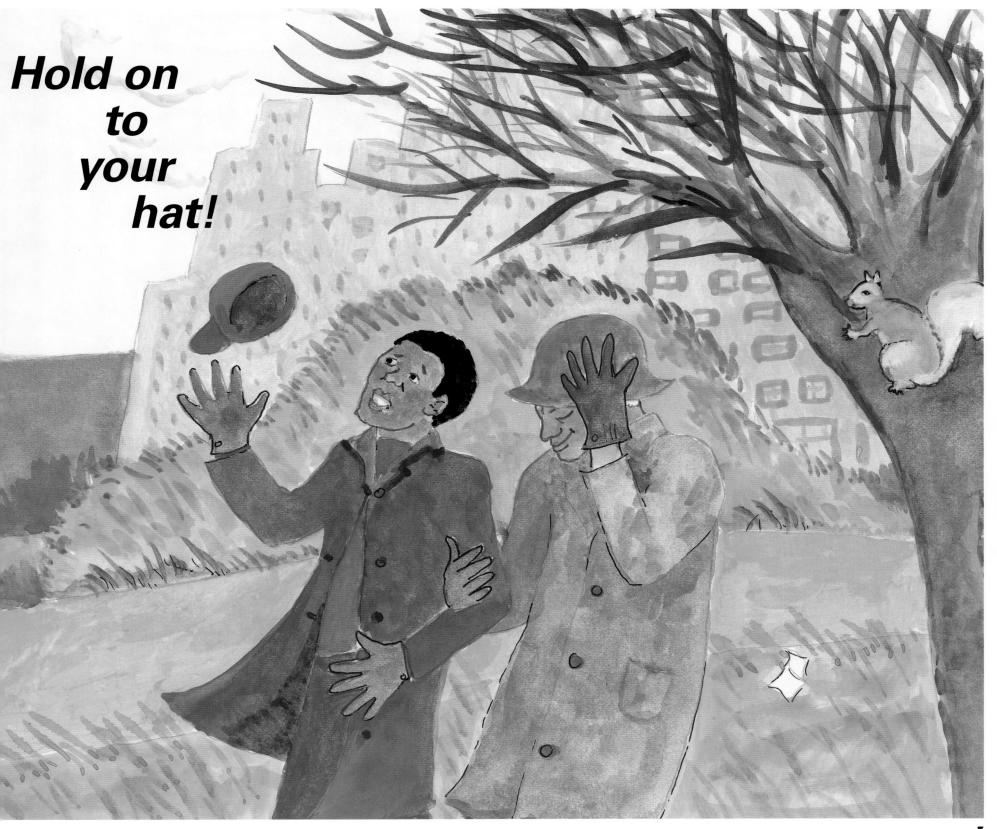

Hold on
to
your
hat!

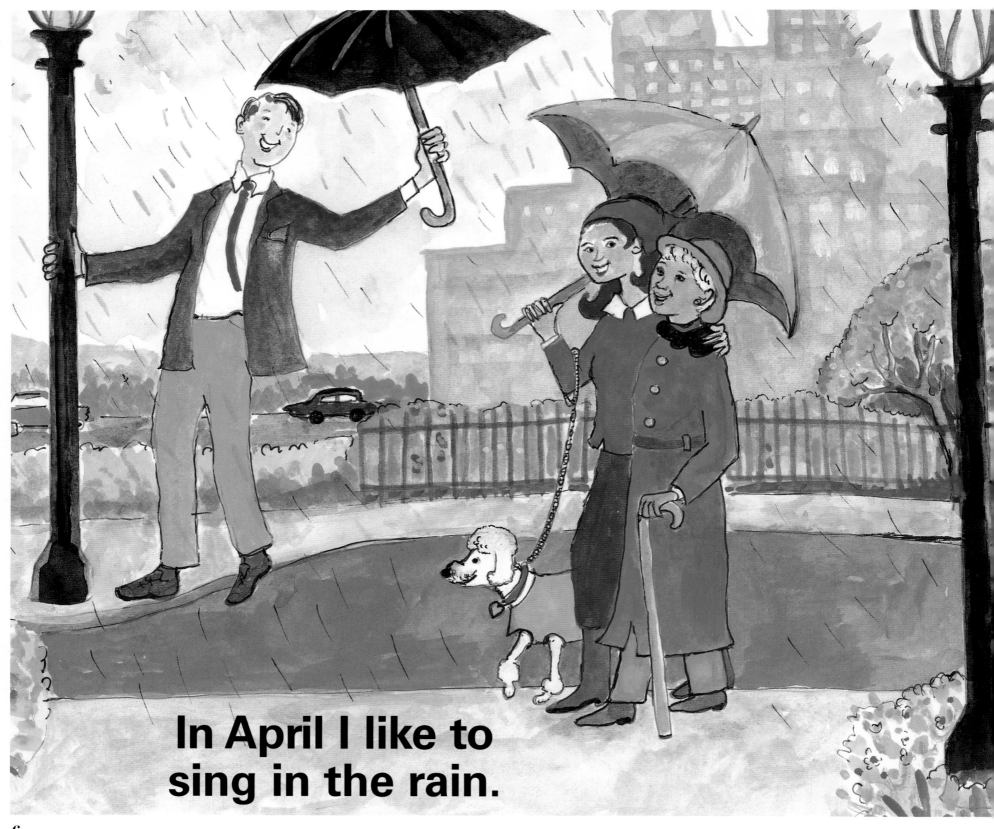

In April I like to sing in the rain.

In May I enjoy all the beautiful flowers.

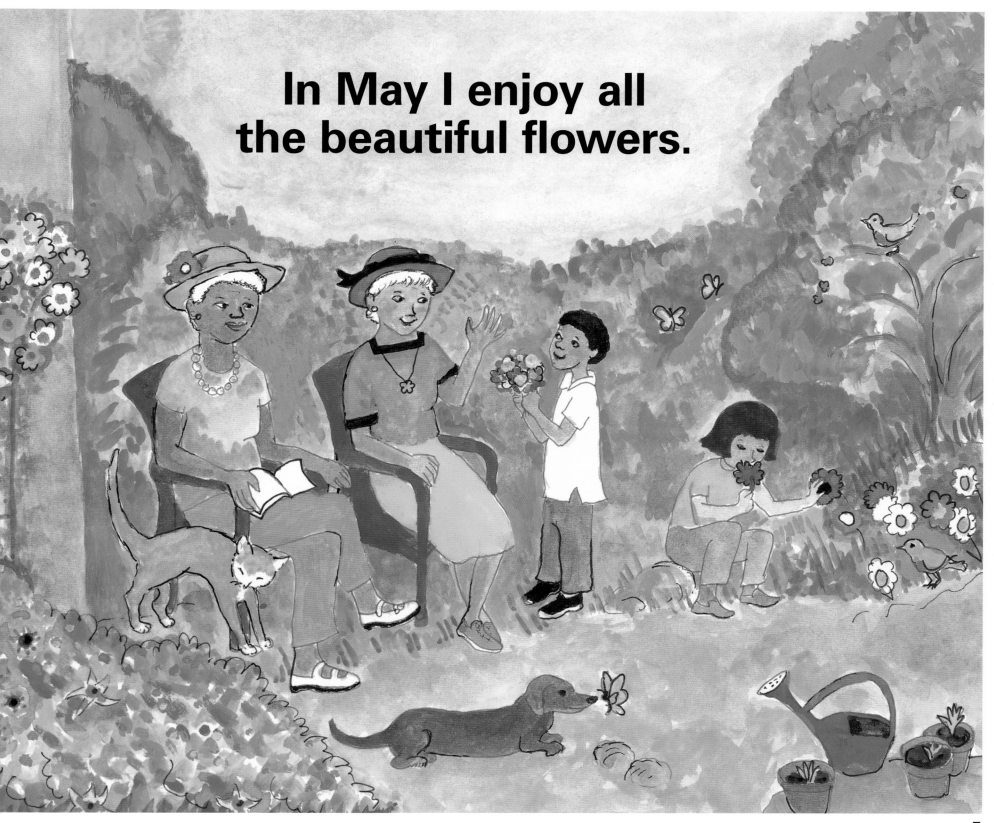

**In June I love going
to weddings—**
*Here comes
the bride!*

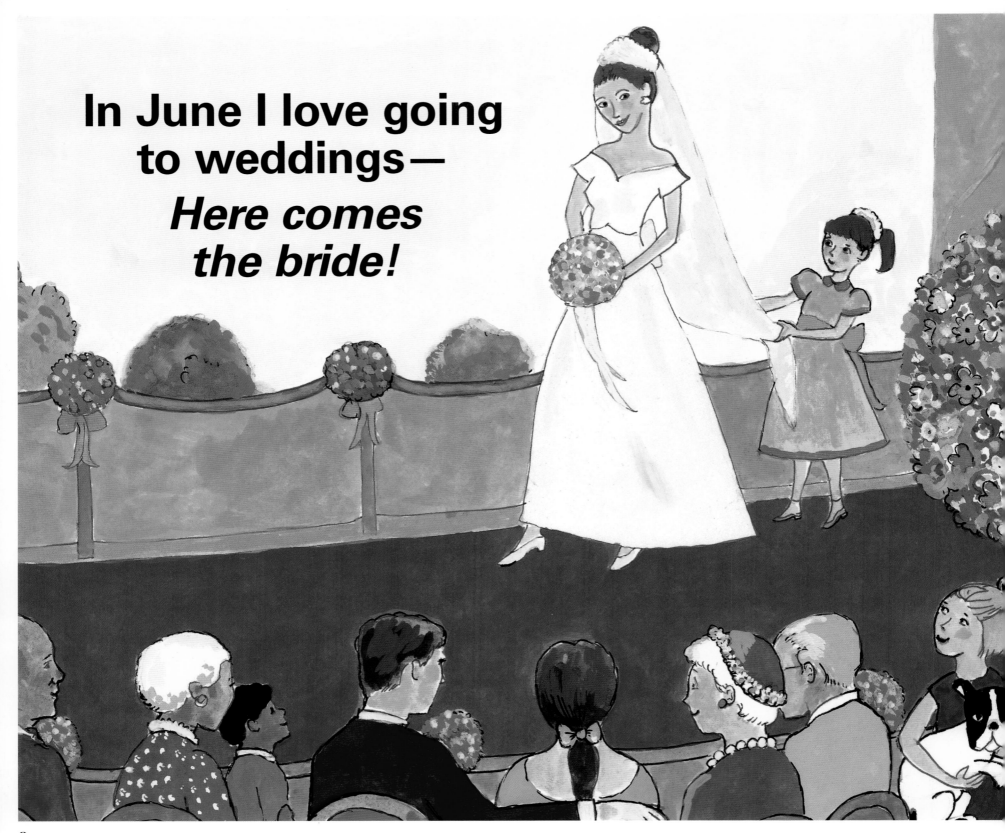

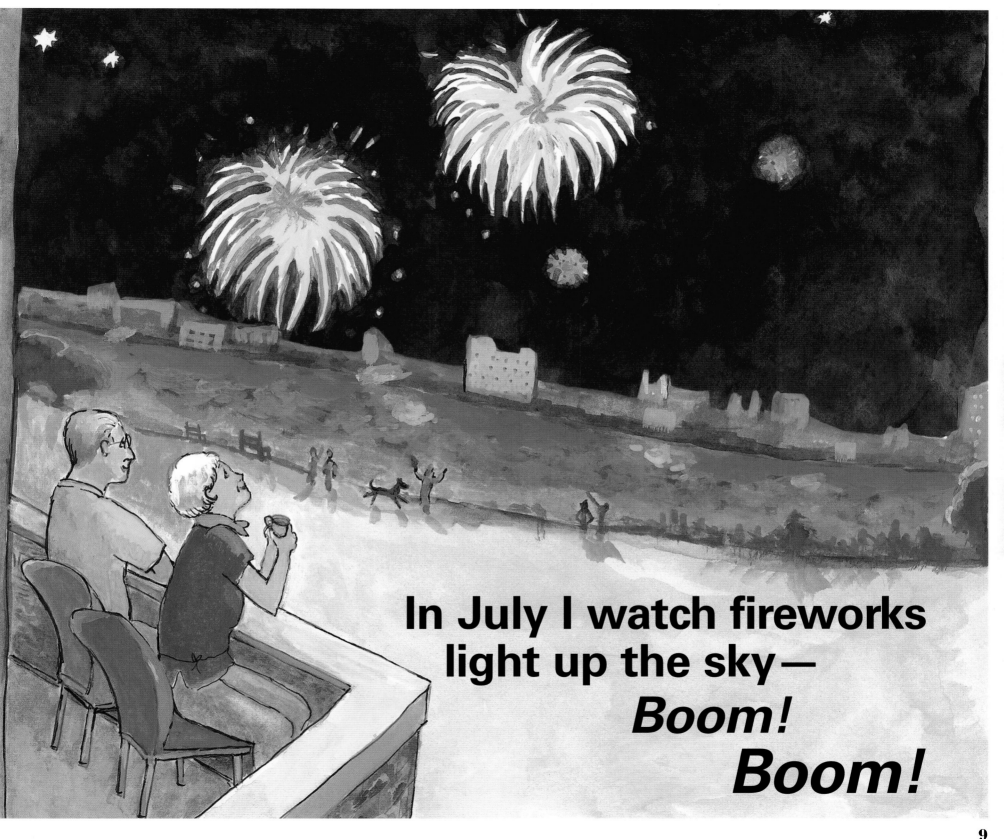

In July I watch fireworks
light up the sky—
> Boom!
>> Boom!

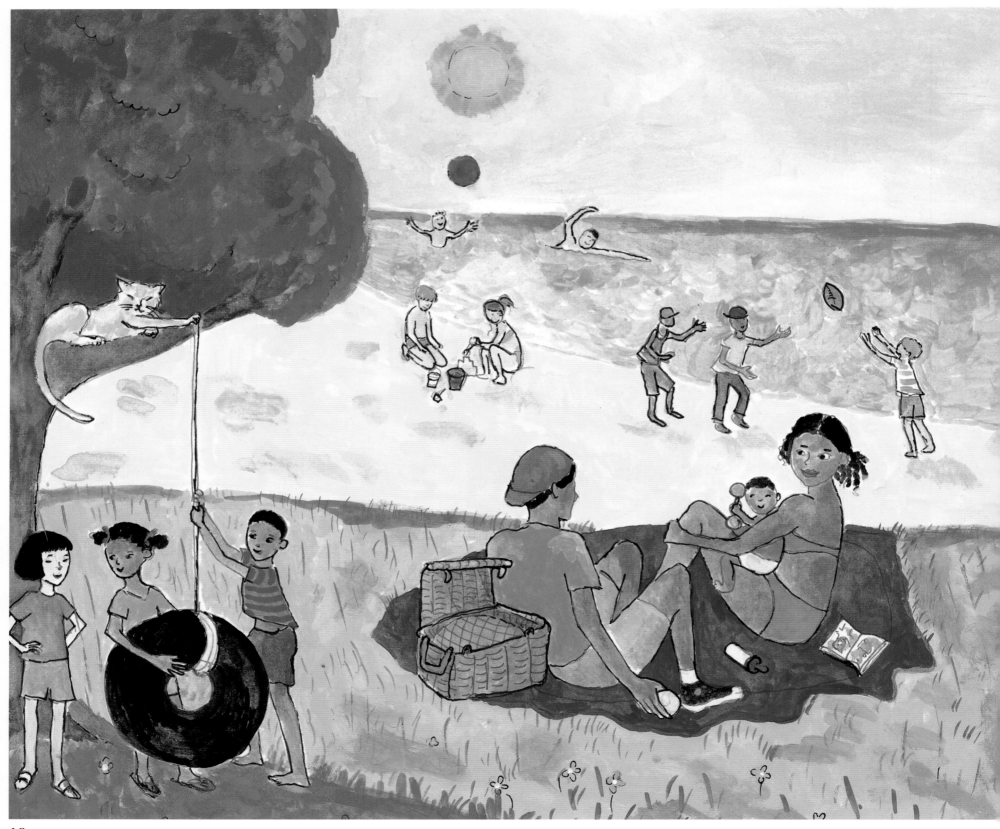

In August
I go on picnics.

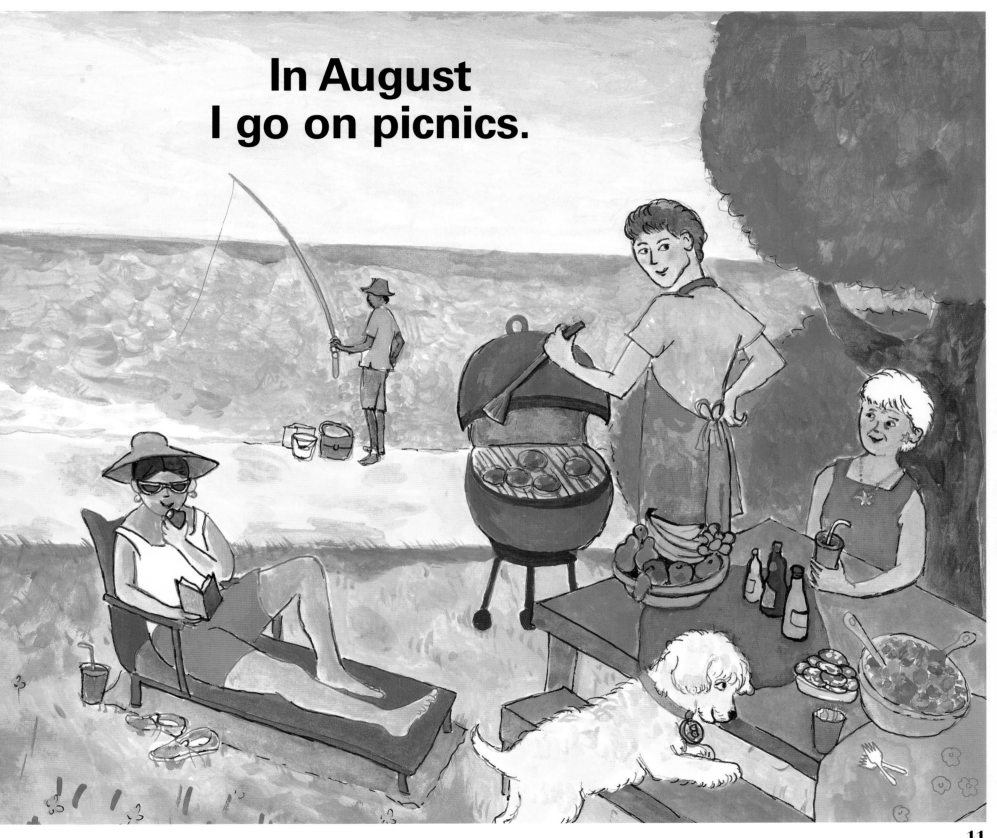

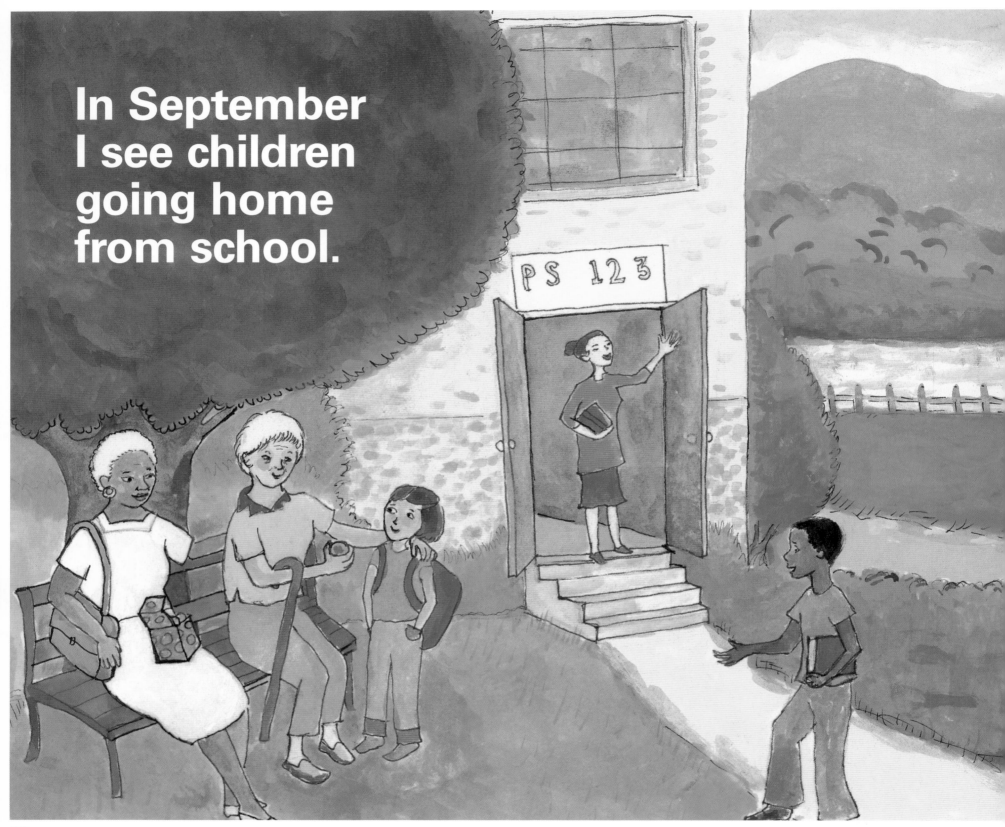

In September
I see children
going home
from school.

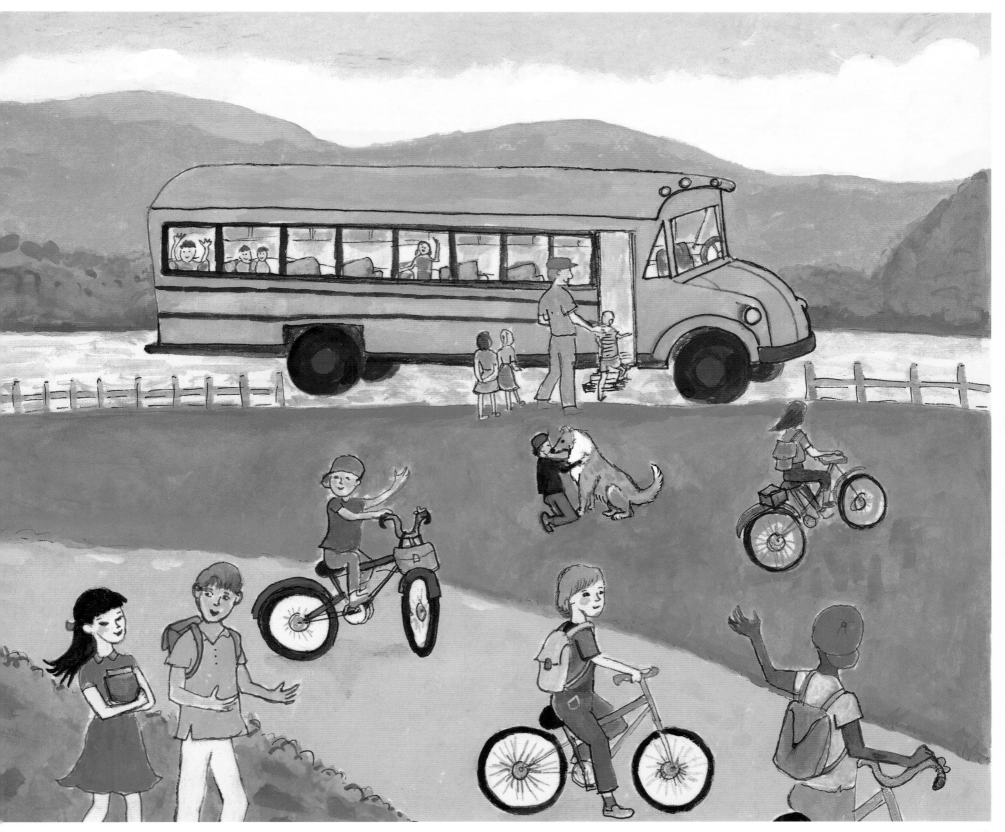

In October I watch the red and yellow leaves fall from the trees.

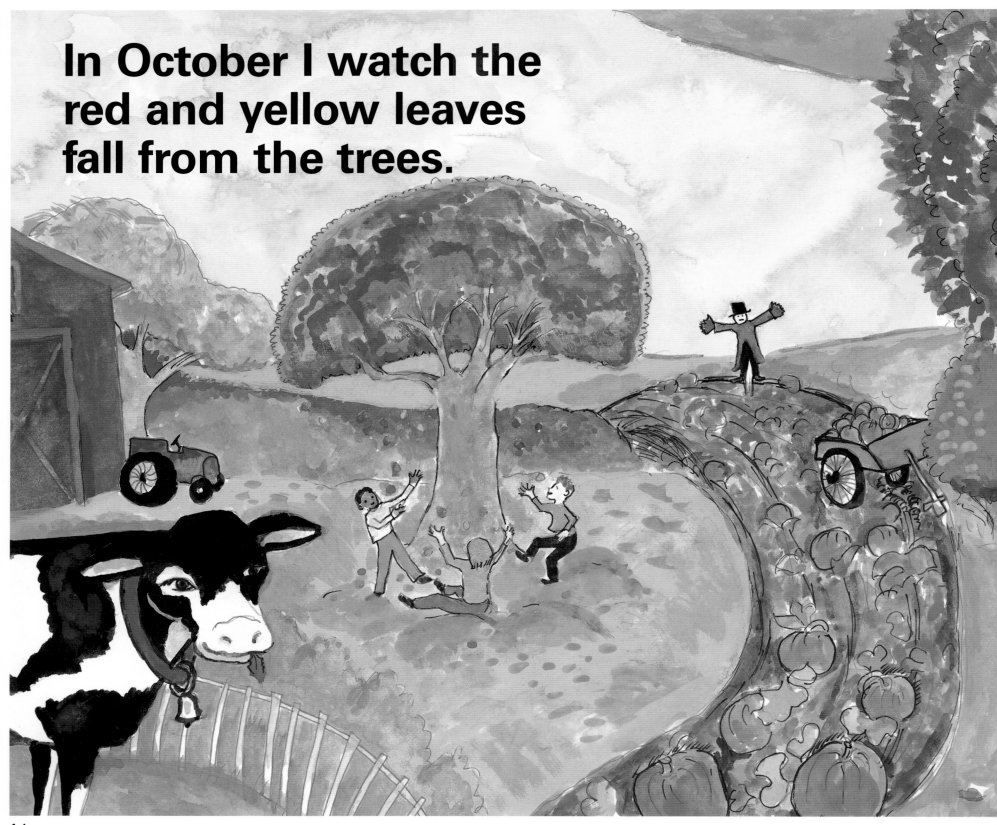

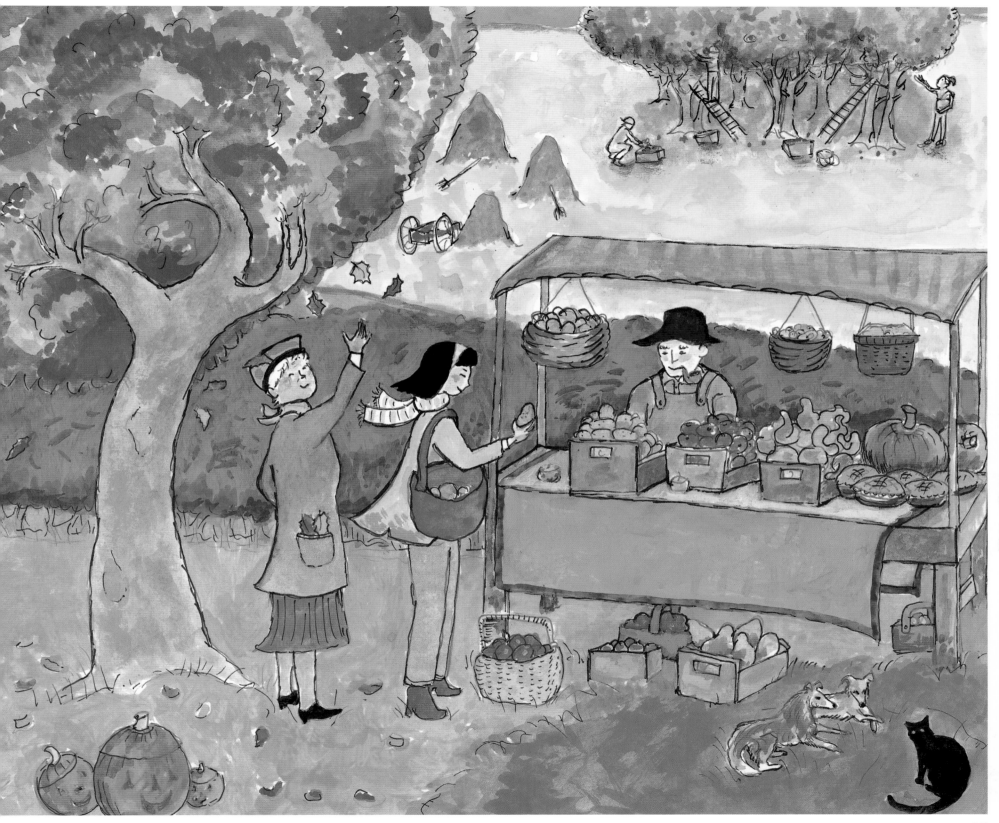

In November I am thankful for so many things.

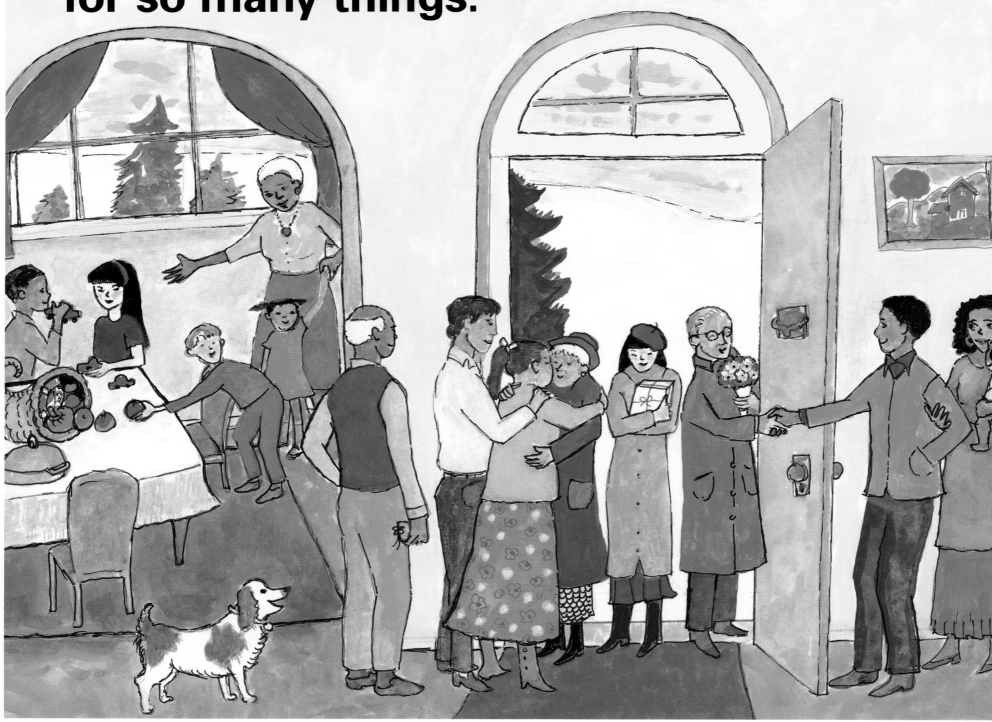

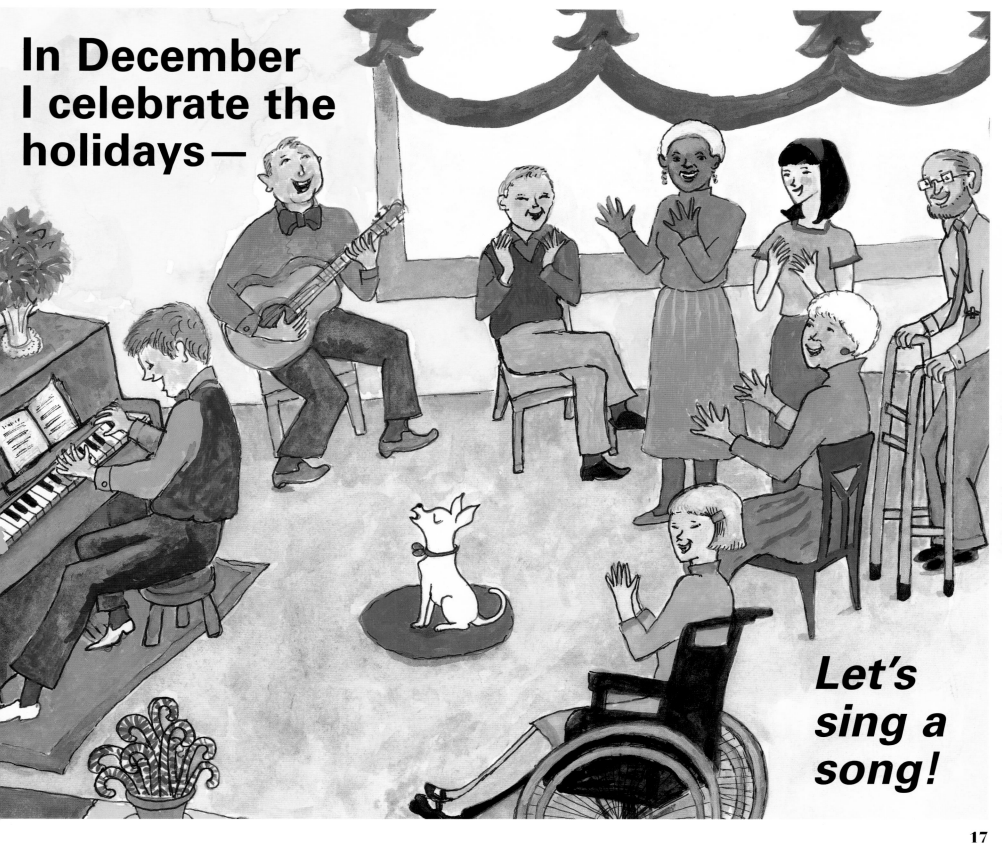

In December
I celebrate the
holidays—

Let's
sing a
song!

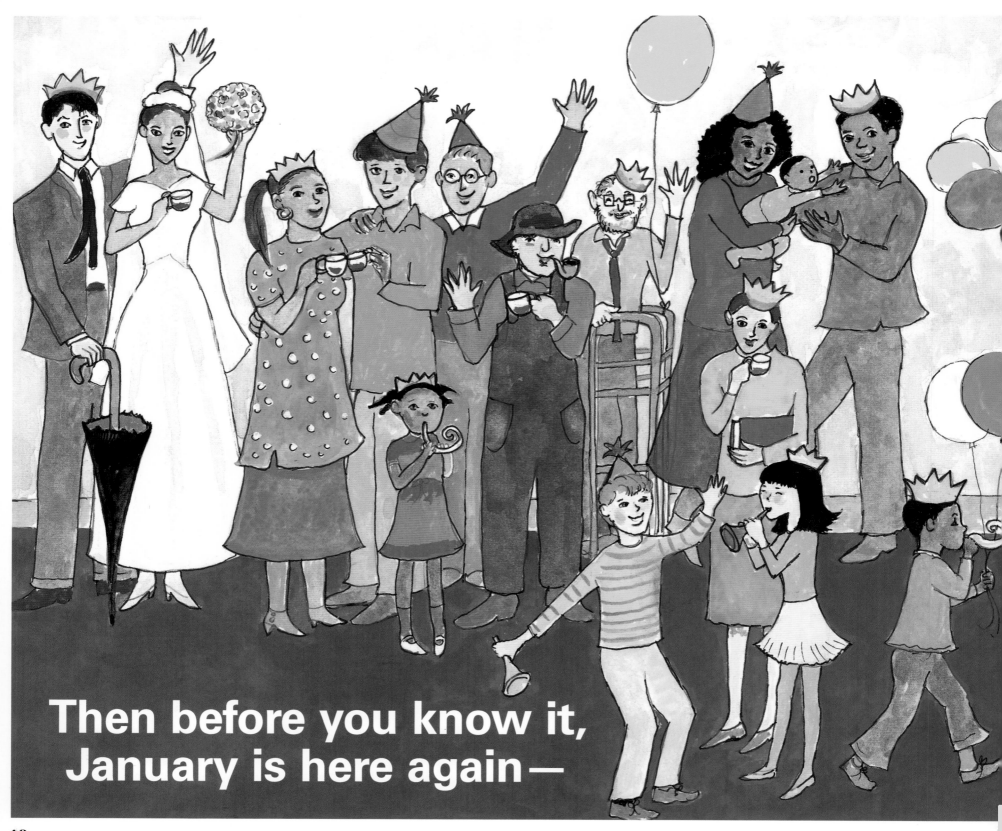

**Then before you know it,
January is here again—**

"Happy New Year to You!"

Sample Conversation Prompts and Songs for Each Page

Page 1   **In January I wish you "Happy New Year!"**

How do you celebrate the new year?
Do you make New Year's resolutions?
What are some things you like about winter?

Songs: *Auld Lang Syne*
        Hail, Hail the Gang's All Here
        Frosty the Snowman
        Let It Snow

Pages 2–3   **In February will you be my Valentine?**

Who would you like to be your Valentine?
How does it feel when you love someone?
Can I give you a hug?

Songs: *I Love You a Bushel and a Peck*
        I Only Have Eyes for You
        I Can't Give You Anything But Love, Baby
        Someone to Watch Over Me
        Some Enchanted Evening

Pages 4–5   **In March I hear the wind blowing through the trees**

How does the wind feel?
What sounds does the wind make?
Do you like to be outside on a windy day?

Songs: *Let's Go Fly a Kite*
        They Call the Wind Maria
        Blow the Man Down
        My Wild Irish Rose

Page 6   **In April I like to sing in the rain**

Do you like to be out in the rain?
Do you like to sing?
What song(s) do you like to sing?

Songs: *Singin' in the Rain*
        Let a Smile Be Your Umbrella
        April Showers
        Somewhere Over the Rainbow

Page 7   **In May I enjoy all the beautiful flowers**

What kind of flowers do you like?
What flowers smell the best?
Did you ever plant flowers or vegetables in a garden?

Songs: *Daisy (A Bicycle Built for Two)*
        Tiptoe Through the Tulips
        I'll Be With You in Apple Blossom Time
        Roses Are Red, Violets Are Blue

Page 8   **In June I love to go to weddings**

Did you get married? What was your wedding like?
What is the best part of being married?
Do you like to dance at weddings? Or right now?

Songs: *Here Comes the Bride*
        Love and Marriage
        You Made Me Love You
        Me and My Gal
        Diamonds Are a Girl's Best Friend

Page 9   **In July I watch fireworks light up the sky**

Do you like to see fireworks?
What sounds do fireworks make?
What do you like about the night sky?

Songs: *Yankee Doodle*
        Twinkle, Twinkle Little Star
        In the Good Old Summertime

Pages 10–11   **In August I go on picnics**

What do you like to eat at a picnic?
What other foods do you like?
Do you like to swim or fish or sail?

Songs: *I Scream, You Scream (We All Scream for Ice Cream!)*
        You Are My Sunshine
        The Ants Go Marching One by One
        My Bonnie Lies Over the Ocean
        Take Me Out to the Ballgame

Pages 12-13   In September I see the children coming home from school

Did you like school?
What did you like to study in school?
What games did you play when you were a child?
How did you get to school? School bus, walk, car?

Songs: *School Days, School Days*
      If You're Happy and You Know It Clap Your Hands
      I Won't Grow Up!
      Playmate Come Out and Play With Me

Pages 14-15   In October I watch the red and yellow leaves fall from the trees

What do you like about the fall season?
Have you ever picked apples from a tree?
What vegetables do you like?
Did you go trick-or-treating at Halloween?

Songs: *Old MacDonald Had a Farm*
      Mairzy Doats
      Don't Sit Under the Apple Tree with Anyone Else But Me
      Ida, Sweet as Apple Cider

Page 16   In November I am thankful for so many things

What are you thankful for?
Who are you thankful for?
Who do you like to visit with?

Songs: *Over the River and Through the Woods*
      Home on the Range
      Home Sweet Home
      They Can't Take That Away From Me

Page 17   In December, I celebrate the holidays

What holidays do you like to celebrate?
What do you like about the holidays?
Are there special holiday foods you like?

Songs: *Jingle Bells*
      Winter Wonderland
      There's No Place Like Home for the Holidays
      With a Song in My Heart

Pages 18-19   Then, before you know it, January is here again

Which is your favorite month?
Did you enjoy reading this book?
Would you like to read this book again? Now? Later?

Songs: *Happy Trails ('Til We Meet Again)*
      Bye Bye Blackbird
      I'll Be Seeing You

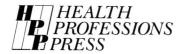

Health Professions Press
Post Office Box 10624
Baltimore, MD 21285-0624
U.S.A.

www.healthpropress.com

The following Two-Lap Book™ is also available from Health Professions Press, Inc.:
The Sunshine on My Face: A Read-Aloud Book for Memory-Challenged Adults.
To order, contact Health Professions Press, Inc. (410-337-9585 or
www.healthpropress.com)

Library of Congress catalog number: RC523.2B873 2006
616.8'3106–dc22
ISBN-13: 978-1-932529-20-3
ISBN-10: 1-932529-20-9

Reinforced library binding. Printed in China.

Illustrated by Jane Freeman.

Two-Lap Books™ are available at a quantity discount with bulk purchases for educational,
therapeutic, and human services programs. For information, please write to: SPECIAL
SALES DEPARTMENT, HEALTH PROFESSIONS PRESS, POST OFFICE BOX 10624,
BALTIMORE, MD 21285 or fax 410-337-8539.

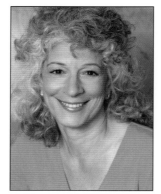

Photograph by Steve Ladner

With a master's degree in Clinical Practices (psychology), **Lydia Burdick's** career has been in human resources. She has been a consultant in an international outplacement firm since 1993. Lydia conceived the idea for her first Two-Lap Book™, *The Sunshine on My Face: A Read-Aloud Book for Memory-Challenged Adults,* in the course of caring for her mother who was diagnosed with Alzheimer's disease. "One of my greatest pleasures," she says, "was sitting next to my mother and hearing her read the words from this book when she had otherwise stopped speaking almost completely."